The Four Cs of Palliative Care: Comfort, Communication, Choices & Control

Basics for Providers & Healthcare Professionals/Clinicians

Nancy Joyner, MS, CNS-BC, APRN, ACHPN®
Palliative Care Clinical Nurse Specialist

NJC
Nancy Joyner
CONSULTING

Disclaimer

This book, *The 4 Cs of Palliative Care: Comfort, Communication, Choices & Control*, addresses perspectives regarding the choice of words and concepts for clinicians, compared to the 2023 GetPalliativeCare.org's website, *Four "C"s Can Help You Understand Palliative Care,"* created for the general public.

Contents

Introduction

The word 'palliative' comes from the Latin word pallium, which means to cloak, cover, protect. When patients receive palliative care, they are cloaked with individualized care as they receive the four Cs: Comfort, Communication, Choices, and Control. The word, 'patient,' comes from the Latin word "patiens, patior," which means to suffer or bear. Thus, palliative care should be provided to all patients. "Palliative care is specialized medical care for people living with a serious illness. This type of care is focused on providing relief from the symptoms and stress of the illness. The goal is to improve quality of life for both the patient and the family" (CAPC website). Palliative care is not based on prognosis or disease but the patient and their "family," improving the quality of life for those with serious illness.

Serious illness is not only about the disease but is a "health condition that carries a high risk of mortality and either negatively impacts a patient's daily function or quality of life or excessively strains the caregiver" (Kelley & Bollens-Lund, 2018). Serious illness may be progressive and irreversible. Healthcare should focus on the human side of care: whatever the person says matters, their function, and quality of life while improving health and decreasing excessive strain and suffering throughout the trajectory of illness (Ballentine, 2018).

Palliative care is a team effort when the four Cs are needed most: comfort, communication, choices, and control. The goal is to improve a patient's quality of life by providing relief from the pain, symptoms, and other stress of serious illness caused by both the disease and the medical treatments. Palliative care provides support. As part of expanding knowledge, please take the time to watch, *Palliative Care: You are a Bridge* (also listed in resources). Doctors, nurses, social workers, chaplains, dietitians, therapists, pharmacists, volunteers, and others are all part of the team, all clinicians working together with the primary care provider and other specialists. Some clinicians are specialized palliative care while others may provide primary palliative care since all clinicians should and do provide some degree of basic palliative care. This type of care is provided at any stage of life and any stage of an illness. It is provided alongside all other appropriate curative treatments.

Palliative care:

- Sees the patient as an individual and who they consider family, as the unit of care
- Pays strict attention to physical, emotional, psychological, social, and spiritual needs
- Uses the interdisciplinary team approach
- Provides ongoing education and support to the patient and family
- Extends across serious illnesses and settings
- Includes anticipatory grief and bereavement support throughout the patient's dying process and death
- Focuses on well-being and manages difficult symptoms (see section: The First C: Comfort. Addresses the everchanging goals of medical care (see section: The Second C: Communication)
- Takes time to help patients and families consider care options and make decisions about quality of life (see section: The Second C: Communication)
- Helps determine when and if to begin, forego or stop treatment/therapy while developing a plan of care (see section: The Third C: Choices)
- Enhances patient and family support by identifying what is important to the patient and family, conveying this to the team, and incorporating to the plan of care (see section: The Fourth C: Control)

Navigating the journey through the health care industry can be so challenging. The paternalism role often seen with clinicians may disrupt the ability for the patient, family, or the clinician to allow patients to make decisions. There is often a sense of urgency and scarcity that does not allow clinicians to connect or build relationships. Palliative care can close the gap within these issues. Palliative care is often confused with hospice. All of hospice is palliative Care, but not all palliative care is hospice. There are similarities and differences. A useful descriptive diagram and distinction flyer that is used: Palliative Care or Hospice? (Developed by ND Palliative Care Taskforce).

The First C: Comfort

(To Comfort Always)

Comfort (Wellbeing)

Today, the word, "comfort" in the medical world is often considered the buzzword for end-of-life and hospice. However, ask any patient for which you are caring if they would want "comfort care while receiving any medical treatment/treatment options," and the answer will be "yes." This statement does not imply no treatment or comfort measures only. The goals of palliative care should lead to the patient's wellbeing and continuously be a priority. Comfort is a multidimensional function, and overall well-being from the perspective of the patient (not the clinicians). Comfort includes all eight aspects (domains) of palliative care as described in the *Clinical Practice Guidelines for Quality Palliative Care* (NCP Guidelines, 2018): 1) structure and processes of care, 2) physical, 3) psychological and psychiatric, 4) social, 5) spiritual, religious and existential, 6) cultural, 7) care for the patient nearing the end of life, and 8) ethical and legal.

According to the NCP Guidelines:

The palliative care interdisciplinary team (IDT) endeavors to relieve suffering and improves quality of life, as defined by the patient and family, through the safe and timely reduction of the physical symptoms and functional impairment associated with serious illness. The goal of symptom management is to improve physical well-being, functionality, and quality of life to a level acceptable to the patient, or to the health care surrogate if the patient is unable to report distress. (p.13).

Serious illness is an important aspect of both the definition and illness trajectories involved with palliative care. Being usually irreversible and progressive, "serious illness is a health condition that carries a high risk of mortality and either negatively impacts a person's daily function or quality of life or excessively strains their caregiver" (Kelly & Bollens-Lund, 2018). The value of serious illness messaging became monumental during COVID-19 and was identified and supported by the John Hartford and Cambia Health Foundation. A website, Serious Illness Messaging, was identified to encourage clinicians to "steal these messages" when explaining Advance Care Planning (ACP), hospice, and palliative care.

According to Coehlo et al., 2016, "Four themes reflect the essence of the lived experience: The Palliative Care, as a response to the patient's needs with advanced disease, attempts to naturalize advanced disease, confrontation with their own vulnerability, openness to the spiritual/spirituality dimension" (p.15). This statement implies comfort to include humanized care environment, symptomatic control, hope, and relationships. Discomfort reflects losses and powerlessness (Coehlo et al, 2016). See the figure below (with permission.

Fig. 1 | From: Comfort experience in palliative care: a phenomenological study

Conceptual representation of the sub-themes and themes base on the findings.

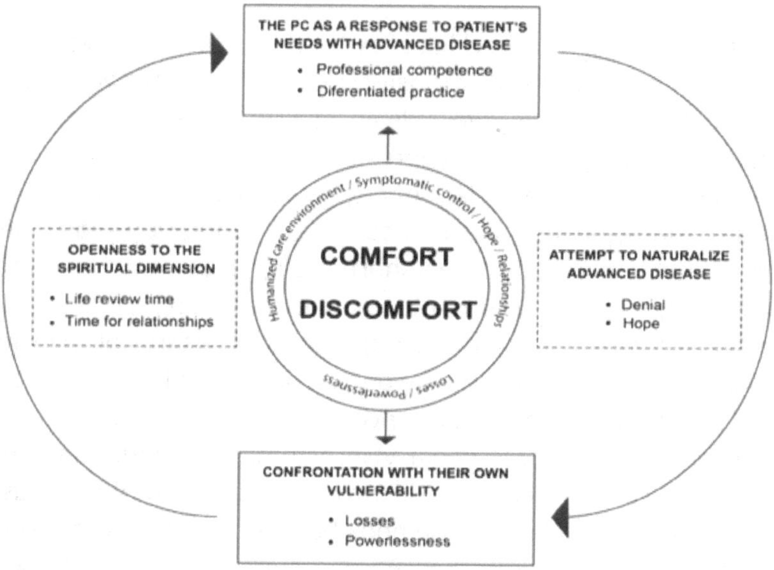

(With permission, Coehlo et al, 2016)

Terminology matters. Pain is truly whatever a patient says it is, since it cannot be measured. As a healthcare team, we often ask on a scale 0-10, but a number is only relevant to gauge the intensity and impact on a patient's quality of life from their perspective, which gives us a baseline to improving comfort. Pain was assigned as the 5th vital sign back in 1996, in an attempt to have it routinely assessed and managed. However, it is not measurable like the other vital signs. After establishing trust and rapport, asking "how are things going?", and "are you comfortable?" prove to be more beneficial. Marsha Farrell's Palliative Pain Primer gives more intensive guidance from the patient's point of view for assessment and management of pain.

Providing comfort and symptom relief goes beyond physical pain. Common symptoms patients experience with serious illness include shortness of breath, nausea, constipation, depression, anxiety, fatigue/loss of energy, drowsiness/tiredness, appetite changes, dry mouth, edema/swelling, weakness, and even hiccups. The Edmonton Symptom Assessment System (ESAS) scale is a great tool to gauge symptoms over time and let others know how a patient is doing. Even the patient themselves can use the tool as well as the family members.

Here is an A through Z Checklist of symptoms to assess beyond pain. Although not necessarily all inclusive, many of these are addressed in the PCNOW Fast Facts (available as an APP) for assessment and management: a) agitation, b) anorexia and cachexia c) anxiety, d) ascites/edema, e) asthenia/lack of energy, f) constipation, g) cough, h) delirium, confusion, terminal restlessness, i) depression, j) diarrhea, k) dry eyes/dry nose, l) dyspnea/shortness of breath, m) dysphagia, n) fatigue, o) fever, p) hiccups, q)nausea and vomiting r) oral secretions- copious, hick, or noisy, s) pruritis, t) seizures or myoclonic jerks, u) skin, wound, malignant wounds, pressure ulcers/Kennedy ulcer, sensitivity, v) sleep disturbance/insomnia/hypersomnia, w) stomatitis, x) weakness/asthenia, y)xerostomia/dry mouth and finally, of course, z) ZZZZZ's (see sleep disturbance/insomnia). Numerous tools and references later in the book have excellent chapters and discussions on these symptoms. Please keep them in your checklist for assessment and management. Patients are reluctant to share information unless they are asked (See Communication section).

Social determinants of health (SDOH) are now becoming a greater focus in the wellbeing for patients. The World Health Organization defines social determinants of health as the "the non-medical factors that influence health outcomes. They are the conditions in which people are born, grow, work, live, and age, and the wider set of forces and systems, shaping the conditions of daily life. The following list provides examples of the social determinants of health that may impact serious illness and can influence health equity in either positive and negative ways include: a) income and social protection, b) education, c) unemployment and job insecurity, d) working life conditions, e) food insecurity, f) housing, basic amenities and the environment, g) social inclusion and non-discrimination, h)structural conflict and i) access to affordable health services of decent quality" (website).

Significant SDOH, affecting palliative care, include transportation, housing, nutrition, social support, caregiver support, economic stability, healthcare access and quality, the physical neighborhood, and community. Childhood experiences, spirituality, income, social status, coping skills, and health behaviors can have direct bearing on a patient's quality of life. These social determinants of health may have a significant impact on the trajectory of person's wellbeing, thus they need to be included in the palliative plan of care for assessment and management (Parker, 2022, 2020).

Although this overview of comfort is brief, the best source of assessing and managing comfort is always the patient and their family. What makes them comfortable? What is comfort to them? Please treat them as if they were your own family.

Key Takeaways

- Clinicians should know how the patient describes comfort and pain whatever it is to them, from baseline to least and most.
- Ongoing assessment and management are provided on all aspects of comfort.
- Family is educated and supported to provide safe/appropriate comfort measures to patient.
- Include the social determinants of health in assessment and plan of care.
- Pain and other symptoms-treating side effects are frequently assessed using best practices.
- Team communicates treatment/therapy alternatives, permitting patient/family to make informed choices.

The Second C: Communication

(conversations/discussions, non-verbal, written, video)

One of the most critical pieces of healthcare is communication. How we present information to patients and their families and what we present can be most valuable or detrimental to the person's life in decision-making. Clinicians often forget (when discussing minor to major objective findings) that medical care has is its own language, is a business, and the knowledge base of the patients may have may only be founded from television, family members, or the internet. Patients may find themselves clueless, almost a blank slate, especially when overwhelmed, in fear, and with extreme apprehension about their future.

Communication comes in different forms. The verbal conversation is often reflective of the clinician's agenda and expectation. The patient may have other things on their mind, fearful to ask questions, and not knowing what to ask. "I don't know what I don't know" is a phrase often used by the individuals and families' clinicians who are caring for their loved one. Clinicians may neglect to ask basic questions, "help me understand" to know where the individual's thoughts and knowledge are at the point of reference. Ask yourself, "what is their agenda?" Remember, not all people communicate or learn the same way. Include handouts, videos, resources, and hands on activities when possible. And don't forget the children.

Once introductions are made, sit down and be at eye level to establish being on their level while demonstrating engagement and concern. Sitting down does not require longer time. Often patients see this effort as caring and offering more time. Do indicate the amount of time you have, even if you are able to finish earlier. Find out more about who they are as a person, what their day is like, their background, their legacy and positive aspects of their life. Starting a conversation can be as easy as asking, "how are things going?" versus "how are you?" where often the answer is 'fine.' Whenever a question is asked, or a new topic explored, remember to allow time for thought and answer or to ask a question. Clinicians are not only in a hurry with constant battle for their time, they are also uncomfortable with silence. Try not speaking for 10 seconds and try not overtalking or interrupting. These are challenges clinicians face every day.

Often neglected in communication is in establishing the patient's aspects of hope. In Steve Pantilat's 2019 MedTalk, he suggests, the golden question is asking, 'when you think about the future, what do you hope for?' If that is what is important, we should do that now. Hope never dies, it changes. Communication should center providing enough time and clarification of the patient's comfort and hope. When a person asks, how long and the clinician's prediction of survival is often less than what is shared with the patient and their family, false hope occurs and may greatly alter the choices a patient makes. Using the Serious Illness Trajectories and other screening tools can aid in more accurate prognosis and probable (expected) outcome. There can negative outcomes for those who are unaware of the progression of their disease and their current status.

Medical care has three key elements: diagnosis, prognosis, and treatment/therapy. Since technology, research, and science have evolved, diagnosis and treatment have become the major focus of clinicians with less focus on prognosis. Although clinicians have disease modification as the primary goal of most encounters, discovering what the patient's goals, wishes, and preferences is essential but often overlooked. Are they included in your personal checklist?

Advance Care Planning (ACP) goals of care planning and talking about the future probable (expected) outcome are key quality communication needs in palliative care. The tools to assist with getting started include The Conversation Project's, "Your Conversation Starter Guide" or "What Matters to Me" Workbook as well as the Go Wish card game. Instead of an office, try sitting down in a quiet room with a table to allow patients and family members to have these often-hard conversations in a more palatable setting. Often, it will take two of more sessions to complete an advance directive/health care directive. There may be times when other team members or ACP facilitators will assist with the completion.

Medical decisions should be based on shared decision-making. Medicine has moved away from the paternalistic attitude of the early to mid-20th century (although many elders still rely on what the clinician or provider recommend). Language should be in terms the patient and family can understand. Someone with medical decision-making capacity must be included, so a three-way conversation is always advised. Having a third person to review and summarize, as well as clarify, is very beneficial. The central focus in palliative care is often the communication of the risks, benefits, burdens, and probable (expected) outcome of treatment/therapy such as tests, surgeries, medications, and disease process.

Often providers will offer treatments that are best suited for others with similar disease, but they neglect to discuss the default policy/standard of care to always provide all life sustaining treatments for any person who has not told by the health care team there are treatments that are not wanted. Some of these may be medically nonbeneficial treatment (futile treatment). Normalize and neutralize the situation to allow a more objective thought process. Remember, you are in their space /their guest, accompanying them on their journey. However, ask permission, ask questions, and don't anticipate what may be said.

Positive impacts of outstanding communication include:

- Accompanying them on their emotional journey, establishing where they are versus what we know
- Building trust/respect
- Establishing what really matters

- Helping clinicians understand
- Creating an atmosphere; When you need us, we will be here.
- Allowing the conversation to put them in control
- Using the team approach; we are in this together.
- Providing hope while providing humility and honesty along the spectrum
- Discussing probability versus possibility of interventions

Key Takeaways

- Allow time and treat patients as humans more than patients when discussing medical issues.
- Always focus on hope for things that are realistic and reasonable (although the patient may not always be at the same understanding or perspective)
- Be sincere and stay engaged
- Offer information in terms that are understand

The Third C: Choices

(focus from the patient's perspective)

With the ever-changing status of health-options, there are endless options and choices for the patient and family to make. However, the probable (expected) outcome/discharge for all medical interventions can be one of three: recovery, dependence, or death. It is often difficult for clinicians, patients, and families to imagine that interventions won't always be beneficial, and patients don't always recover. From the moment a patient walks into a clinic or hospital, these probable outcomes may be foremost in their thoughts.

The decision to start or stop life-sustaining treatments can be both ethically and emotionally challenging to everyone involved. However, since the 1990 Patient Self-Determination Act and the principle of patient autonomy gives every patient who has medical decision-making capacity regarding their current health status and choices, the right to decline any medical intervention or to ask that a treatment be stopped. This right applies even when that decision is expected to lead to their death and regardless of whether the patient is terminally ill. When a patient lacks appropriate capacity, the patient's surrogate/proxy/health care agent may decline treatment or ask that an intervention be stopped in keeping with legal and ethical aspects of the surrogate decision-maker. When an intervention no longer helps to achieve the patients' goals for care or desired HRQOL: Quality of Life it is ethically appropriate for clinicians to withdraw it.

Reassuring patients that they are making right choices for themselves by approaching the decisions appropriately will often ease their stress and anxiety. Adding new tools, choices, and alternatives will provide hope in a more meaningful way than to have patients feel they have "given up," "pulling the plug," "being a burden," or being abandoned. Good communication to lower the uncertainty may help to mitigate these difficulties to some degree. Discontinuing, withholding, and withdrawing are difficult terms for everyone involved. Easy solutions, such as time-limited trials, with goals and the time to review should be offered. Often neglected is the choice to opt-out with alternatives, which should be offered and explored.

DNR does not mean Do Not Treat! Even the choice to forego CPR attempts and Allow Natural Death (A.N.D.) should not influence the choice of treatment/therapy or the clinician's understanding of the goals of care. Often, the patient is hoping for a cure and anticipating recovery or reversible outcomes. This situation happens frequently with a combination of missed or clarifying communication and expectations of hope. The decision made to forego treatments often comes after time limited trials; treatment/therapy options including to opt-out need to be offered.

Discontinuing, withholding, and withdrawing are difficult terms for everyone involved.

Once a decision has been made to either withhold or withdraw treatment/therapy, a well-defined explanation of what the patient and family should expect, what are the next steps, what they may see, and some aspect of timeframes may ease some of the fear of the unknown. The risks, benefits, burdens, and probable (expected) outcomes need to be discussed.

Here are examples of some of the choices patients and families must make:

- Hospitalization
- Tests and procedures
- Infusions/medications
- Antibiotics (oral or IV)
- Surgery
- Life Sustaining Treatment

- CPR/Code Status (one of two choices: Attempt or Allow Natural Death (A.N.D.)
- -
- Respiratory support
  - » Oxygen therapy
  - » BiPAP/CPAP
  - » Intubation/Mechanical ventilation
  - » Tracheostomy
- Cardiac treatments
  - » Cardiac Catheterization
  - » Bypass surgery
  - » Pacemaker/Defibrillator
  - » Dialysis
  - » Rehabilitation
  - » Long Term Care/Skilled Nursing
  - » Assisted Living

Please humanize discussions, regarding choices. They are often infused with emotion, concern, grief, anger, disbelief, and frustration. Consider how you would discuss these with your own family before approaching these topics with the patients and family for whom you care.

Key takeaways

- Provide the time-limited option with goals of the treatment/ therapy, a check-in date, and plans if it doesn't meet the goals.
- Provide the option to opt-out with what can be done, instead, to provide comfort and quality

Remember, DNR does not mean Do Not Treat.

The Fourth C: Control

(care coordination, collaborative care)

For patients to have control, the medical team must employ care coordination and collaborative care. Care coordination involves the team working together with other clinicians and community service providers, supporting the continuity of care across the illness trajectory, and all settings, especially during transitions of care. The team uses processes to ensure access, quality, and continuity of care. Care coordination includes carefully organizing patient care activities and sharing information with all of the team concerned with a patient's care to achieve safer and more effective care. "This [statement] means that the patient's needs and preferences are known ahead of time and communicated at the right time to the right people, and this information is used to provide safe, appropriate, and effective care to the patient (Agency for Healthcare Research and Quality (AHRQ), 2018) ."

Collaborative care is stressed in the AMA Code of Ethics. Collaboration involves the interdisciplinary team's focus on the patient's needs from the perspective of the healthcare team's specialty. " Such teams are defined by their dedication to providing patient-centered care, protecting the integrity of the patient-physician relationship, sharing mutual respect and trust, communicating effectively, sharing accountability and responsibility, and upholding common ethical values as team members" (AMA, Code of Medical Ethics, 2001) .

Control rests in the patient's choices, preferences, and wishes. Value-based care and prioritizing patient outcomes are becoming the driving force for medical care in the United States with the push from the payers. Although there is much resistance to change, one of the rewarding aspects of palliative care is that the patient and family have always been the focus. The patient is in control and the central focus, when it comes to palliative care. Some patients accept this willingly, some oppose this role, and others use it to their advantage. Cultural aspects are often considered with relevancy to patient-centered care.

Expressed examples of patient-centered care and control by the patient include:

- Being treated with dignity and respect
- Treating family with dignity and respect
- Relieving burdens on the family
- Achieving pain and symptom management control to their level of comfort
- Avoiding the financial burdens of other
- Preventing any dependence on others
- Achieving a sense of control
- Strengthening relationships with loved ones
- Desiring to follow family's preferences (whatever the family says)
- Following religious teachings
- Living as long as possible (but defining what 'living' means to the patient)
- Avoiding inappropriate prolongation of the dying process
- Wishing for a dignified death
- Achieving emotional well-being
- Feeling life has completion
- Obtaining overall well-being for them and their family
- Addressing needs of the person's unique spiritual/spirituality

- Honoring treatment/therapy preferences
- Having a functional and healthy relationship with the health care team

Family's wishes:

- Having their loved one's wishes honored
- Being included in the decision processes
- Providing support and assistance at home
- Offering practical help (transportation, medicines, equipment)
- Educating on personal care needs (bathing, feeding, toileting)
- Delivering honest information
- Having 24/7 access to talk to someone
- Having privacy with their loved one
- Being listened to
- Being remembered and contacted after the death

Besides ACP conversations and completing advance directives, clinicians have the POLST paradigm, conversation, and form to use to honor a patient's wishes, regarding life sustaining treatment. POLST is recognized in some form, even by different names, in all 50 states and some parts of Canada. Please visit your state's POLST program and reach out to the coordinator.

Key takeaways

- Palliative Care's priority should always be individually focused for each patient, including the family.
- Giving the patient control is paramount to quality care.
- Respecting the patient with each encounter.
- Utilizing POLST to honor the individual's wishes, regarding life sustaining treatment.

Conclusion

The 4 Cs of Palliative Care: Comfort, Communication, Choices, and Control need to be incorporated into the healthcare for all people, facing serious illness. The evidence-based research presented in this booklet provides support for clinicians to implement the 4Cs into their daily practice. In addition, the glossary helps clarify the distinction among the various terms used in this booklet. Understanding the terminology will also help clinicians explain and interpret the medical terminology to seriously ill patients. Quality, competent, and compassionate care for seriously ill people ,utilizing the 4Cs, is the ultimate goal of this booklet.

Serious Illness Case Study

Patty Smith is a 70-year-old lady admitted with severe abdominal pain, weakness, hypotension, hypoxia, and elevated WBC. Her past medical history includes Type 2 Diabetes Mellitus with moderate diabetic polyneuropathy, hypertensive diabetic chronic kidney disease, stage 3, primary osteoarthritis, history of Transient Ischemic Attack (TIA) and cerebral infarction without residual deficits.

Vital signs remained abnormal. She was admitted to the hospital since her vitals, lab values, and symptoms were not stabilizing. An abdominal CT scan was done, which showed evidence of an abdominal mass. An ultrasound technician came into Patty's room, brought his equipment, and placed it next to her bed. He said he had come in to do an ultrasound through her vagina, ordered by the physician. Patty said she didn't know this test was going to be done or why he was doing it. The technician explained to her that the doctor had ordered it, so he was going to perform this ultrasound. He started the procedure and placed the probe into her vagina, trying to open her cervix. It was so painful to Patty that she cried out in pain and was actually screaming.

The charge nurse came in find out what was going on. Patty explained that it was so traumatic for her and how she had told the technician not to do it, but he said that the doctor had ordered it and just continued with the procedure. The charge nurse talked to Patty, then she talked to the technician and told him to stop. Patty was relieved the charge nurse advocated for her and had the procedure stopped. All 4 Cs were overlooked in this case study.

- Patty was experiencing severe physical pain as well as emotional and psychological trauma and discomfort. In this example, when the charge nurse said to stop, it allowed her to relax and feel very comforted that someone was listening to what Patty was saying, telling her and the technician. Stopping also relieved the acute physical discomfort.
- Lack of communication was evident. Patty did not know why or what was happening. She did not know why the test was ordered. When he started doing the actual ultrasound and Patty was in extreme pain, she was so anxious because of the lack of communication between the doctor who ordered it, the technician and herself. The technician was very embarrassed because he was causing me pain; but he insisted since it was ordered, he had to do it.
- Patty was not given any choice to have this procedure done, including the the risks, benefits, or pain that could accompany the procedure. She was not even given the choice to stop and forego the procedure.
- Patty was not allowed to say no to a procedure that was causing physical and emotional pain and discomfort.

Recommendations

The following recommendations for clinicians comes from Patty and years of practice, feedback, and research on palliative care:

- **Comfort:** Make it first priority. "How are things going?" is a good beginning. It is hard to have communication, make choices, or be in control without every element of comfort being explored.
- **Communication:** Provide someone to interpret the medical jargon into plain English to every patient, especially those with serious illness, undergoing procedures and tests that may not be fully understood.
- **Choices:** Discuss with patients what tests will be ordered and why they are being done. Explain what results for which they are looking, why they're using those particular tests, the risks, benefits, and probable (expected) outcome. Allow the patient to opt-out or do a time-limited treatment if possible.
- **Control:** Allow the patients some control over what tests are being ordered and what is ahead. Provide necessary patient education as well as support.

Glossary/Definition of Terms

Advance Care Planning (ACP)
"Advance care planning is a process that supports adults at any age or stage of health in understanding and sharing their personal values, life goals, and preferences regarding future medical care. The goal of advance care planning is to help ensure that people receive medical care that is consistent with their values, goals, and preferences during serious and chronic illness" (Sudore et al, 2017).

advance directive/health care directive
Known by other names, is "a legal document that states a person's wishes about receiving medical care if that person is no longer able to make medical decisions because of a serious illness or injury" (National Cancer Institute, n.d., para.1).

Allow Natural Death (A.N.D.)
A medical order that ensures aggressive comfort measures are provided and acknowledges that the person is dying. The choice to forgo life-extending treatments, such as cardiopulmonary resuscitation, when the person is actively dying (Palliledia, 2022).

capacity vs competency
"Capacity is a functional assessment and a clinical determination about a specific decision that can be made by any clinician familiar with a patient's case... Competency is a global assessment and legal determination made by a judge in court" (Odden & Dastidar, 2011).

care
(vs caring): "TAKING CARE OF PATIENTS emphasizes objective, professional care, such as the medical and psychological aspects of nursing. CARING FOR PATIENTS, on the other hand, is a humanistic

way of interacting with patients that demonstrates sincere care and concern for patients simply because they are human beings" (Paulson, 2004, Abstract).

care coordination
"Care coordination is the deliberate organization of patient care activities between two or more participants (including the patient) involved in a patient's care to facilitate the appropriate delivery of health care services. Organizing care involves the marshalling of personnel and other resources needed to carry out all required patient care activities and is often managed by the exchange of information among participants responsible for different aspects of care" (NCHPC-NCP Guidelines, 2019, p. 60).

choices
Healthcare professionals are expected to offer choices, which promote and enhance autonomy and be beneficial, which is the right thing to do. Choices offered come with responsibility and decision-making, which usually impact individuals and the outcomes that can be achieved (Zolkefi, 2017).

clinician (healthcare professional)
"Any health professional providing direct care to a person and their families, whether primary care practitioners or specialist consultants." (National Consensus Project's Clinical Practice Guidelines for Quality Palliative Care (NCP Guidelines), 2018).

code status
Resuscitation orders. What we should or shouldn't do if the person's heart stopped beating, separate from all other life-sustaining treatments (Goldish & Rosielle, 2018).

collaborative care
"In health care, teams that collaborate effectively can enhance the quality of care for individual patients. By being prudent stewards and delivering care efficiently, teams also have the potential to expand access to care for populations of patients. Such teams are defined by their dedication to providing patient-centered care, protecting the integrity of the patient-physician relationship, sharing mutual respect and trust, communicating effectively, sharing accountability

and responsibility, and upholding common ethical values as team members" (AMA, Code of Medical Ethics, 2001).

comfort

"Humanized care, differentiated environment, symptomatic control, hope, and relationships. The discomfort emerges from the losses and powerlessness against their situation" (Coelho et al., 2016).

comfort care

The most basic palliative care interventions that provide immediate relief of symptoms, "dangerous misconception that clinical care is binary and that patients must choose between focusing on comfort or not" (Pottash, 2019).

comfort measures only

"Comfort Measures Only refers to medical treatment of a dying person where the natural dying process is permitted to occur while assuring maximum comfort. It includes attention to the psychological and spiritual/spirituality needs of the patient and support for both the dying patient and the patient's family. Comfort Measures Only is commonly referred to as "comfort care" by the general public. It is not equivalent to a physician order to withhold emergency resuscitative measures, such as Do Not Resuscitate (DNR)" (Joint Commission National Quality Measures, 2018, para.1: Definition).

communication

"Promoting and facilitating open communication to foster patient- and family-centered shared decision-making, and advance care planning is essential. Ethnic and cultural differences should be acknowledged. Family members' decision-making strategies around options of care, location, and preferences should take into account cultural, ethnic, and religious preferences. The earlier these discussions can occur, the better, so when there are unexpected changes in a patient's condition, discussions have already happened, and decisions have been made" (2018 NCP guidelines, 2018, p. 61; Given & Reinard, 2017).

control

(Patient in control/Patient-centered care) "Patient- and family-centered care encourages the active collaboration and shared decision-making between patients, families, and providers to design and manage a customized and comprehensive care plan" (NEJM Catalyst, 2017).

cure
"A subset of treatments that reverse illnesses completely or end medical problems permanently" (Pallipedia, 2022).

default policy/standard of care
"Everyone receives the standard of care during a medical emergency (when you cannot communicate)—unless they have a legal document or medical order to direct health care providers to direct them otherwise" (Understanding Advance Care Planning, National POLST, 2022).

dependence
(opposite of independence) *the state of relying on or needing someone or something for aid, support* to sustain function and health due to loss of function (physical, mental capacity, etc.).

diagnosis
"The process of identifying a disease, condition, or injury from its signs and symptoms. A health history, physical exam, and tests, such as blood tests, imaging tests, and biopsies, may be used to help make a diagnosis" (National Cancer Institute, n.d., para.1).

discomfort
"can be physical or psychological and is characterized by an unpleasant feeling, resulting in a natural response of avoidance or reduction of the source of the discomfort. Pain is one of the causes for discomfort, but not every discomfort can be attributed to pain" (Ashkenazy & DeKeyser Ganz, 2019).

DNR does not mean Do Not Treat
DNR does not entail a preference against other invasive treatments. It requires a conversation as "some studies have indicated that the presence of the DNR or DNI itself increases death rates, unrelated to a disease or trauma" (Baktari, 2021).

Edmonton Symptom Assessment System (ESAS)
The ESAS was developed as a simple, easy-to-use symptom screening tool, which ideally needs to be integrated within an in-depth clinical interview process. Its focus is on a single dimension of symptom assessment (i.e. severity) with nine common symptoms (Edmonton Symptom Assessment System – Revised (ESAS-r) A. (Bruera et. al., 1991; AHS Edmonton Zone Palliative Care Program, CH Palliative Institute & University of Alberta, 2019)

end-of-life
It begins the minute we are born. However, "the period when death is imminent, and life expectancy is limited to a short number of hours or days. The term has been used to describe the last 12 months of life" (Pallipedia, 2022).

family
Always defined by the individual who constitutes their family and how they will participate in care and decision-making. (Institute for Patient- and Family-Centered Care (IPFCC, n.d.).

goals of care
"A process between provider and patient that is repeated, and which involves assessing the patient's hopes, fears, worries, and sense of purpose through illness. Goal-concordant care has been suggested as clinical care that helps a patient reach an identifiable goal, while respecting treatment preferences or limitations the patient has placed on their clinical care" (Pallipedia, 2022).

health care
"Health care is a fundamental human good because it affects our opportunity to pursue life goals, reduces our pain and suffering, helps prevent premature loss of life, and provides information needed to plan for our lives. Society has an obligation to make access to an adequate level of care available to all its members, regardless of ability to pay" (AMA Code of Medical Ethics, 2022).

health care professional
See clinician (healthcare professional)

healthcare provider
See provider

HRQOL: Quality of Life
Quality of life (QOL) is a broad multidimensional that includes domains related to physical, mental, emotional, and social functioning and usually includes subjective evaluations of both positive and negative aspects of life. HRQOL are those aspects of overall quality of life that can be clearly shown to affect health—either physical or mental. It is an individual's or a group's perceived physical and mental health over time. (CDC, Healthy People 2020, Davis & Hui, 2017, Pallipedia)

hope
"A multidimensional dynamic force that is characterized by a confident, yet uncertain expectation of achieving something good, which is realistically possible and personally significant" (Pallipedia, 2022).

hospice
Medical care for people with an anticipated life expectancy of 6 months or less when medical focus shifts to symptom management and quality of life. (Hospice Foundation of America, n.d.)

patient
The individual patient, resident, client- whomever is being provided health care, in whatever setting.

medical care
"The diagnosis, cure, mitigation, treatment, or prevention of disease; services and supplies applied for the purpose of affecting any structure or function of the body."(Law Insider, n.d.) " The quality of medical care is the degree to which health services for individuals and populations increase the likelihood of desired health outcomes and are consistent with current professional knowledge. Quality of care is that component of the difference between efficacy and effectiveness that can be attributed to care providers, taking account of the environment in which they work.(Pallipedia, 2022). "Standard medical care is treatment that is accepted by medical experts as a proper treatment for a certain type of disease and that is widely used by healthcare professionals. Also called best practice, standard of care, and standard therapy." (National Cancer Institute, n.d.)

medical decision-making capacity
"The ability of a patient to understand the benefits and risks of, and the alternatives to, a proposed treatment or intervention (including no treatment). Capacity is the basis of informed consent" (Barstow, Shahan & Roberts, 2018).

medical treatment/treatment options
"The management and care of a patient for the purpose of combating disease, injury, or disorder. Restrictions on activities are not considered treatment unless the primary purpose of the restrictions is to improve the worker's condition through conservative care. (Law Insider, n.d.). A treatment may be beneficial if it relieves suffering, restores functioning, or enhances the quality of life. The same treatment can be considered burdensome if it causes pain, prolongs the dying process without offering benefit, or adds to the perception of a diminished quality of life. A person's decision to decline life support is deeply personal. (Cleveland Clinic, n.d.)

medically nonbeneficial treatment (futile treatment)
"Medical treatment that has no realistic chance of providing a therapeutic benefit that the patient has the capacity to perceive or appreciate, such as merely preserving the physiologic functions of a permanently unconscious patient or has no realistic chance of returning the patient to a level of health that permits survival without acute level of care or hospital setting" (Nelson & Nazareth, 2013).

recovery
Restoring health and strength after an illness when the illness is reversible.

pain
"Pain is whatever the experiencing person says it is, existing whenever the experiencing person says it does" (McCaffery, 1968) It a common, multi-dimensional symptom, which compromises quality of life for many patients with serious illness. It cannot be measured or compared as the experience of pain varies from one person to the next (Fast Fact #417). "The 2020 revised definition of pain is: 'An unpleasant sensory and emotional experience associated with, or resembling that associated with, actual or potential tissue damage," and is expanded upon by the addition of six key notes and the

etymology of the word pain for further valuable context: 1) Pain is always a personal experience that is influenced to varying degrees by biological, psychological, and social factors; 2) Pain and nociception are different phenomena; 3) Pain cannot be inferred solely from activity in sensory neurons; 4) Through their life experiences, individuals learn the concept of pain; 5) A person's report of an experience as pain should be respected; and 6) Although pain usually serves an adaptive role, it may have adverse effects on function and social and psychological well-being.(IASP Task Force, 2020)

palliative care
"Palliative care is specialized medical care for people with serious illnesses (not based on prognosis). It is appropriate at any age at any stage of a serious illness and can be provided together with curative treatment. Palliative care promotes quality of life by addressing the physical, psychological, emotional, cultural, social, and spiritual needs of patients and families" (CAPC, North Dakota Palliative Care Task Force, 2023).

primary palliative care
(Also known as generalist) "Palliative care that is delivered by health care professionals who are not palliative care specialists, such as primary care clinicians; physicians who are disease-oriented specialists (such as oncologists and cardiologists); and nurses, social workers, pharmacists, chaplains, and others who care for this population but are not certified in palliative care."(NCP Guidelines, 2018, p.64)

POLST
The national term for portable medical orders for those individuals facing seriously illness or frailty. It is part of advance care planning that includes conversation with health care professional about diagnosis, prognosis, treatment options, including time limited-trial or opting out. The outcome is the medical order form, known at the POLST form that travels across settings (National POLST, 2022).

probable (expected) outcome
With all things considered, the consequence of implementing specific interventions (or not intervening), based on the person's individual medical status, other co-morbidities, trajectories, other

tests, clinician's estimate of prognosis, and not based on false hope or possibility. Similar to prognosis but future outlook includes all dimensions of the individual's medical, physical, psychological, emotional and spiritual condition (Pantilat, TEDMED, 2018).

prognosis
"A prediction of the probable outcome of a disease based on an individual's condition and the usual course of the disease as seen in similar situations." (Pallipedia, 2022). Note probable, not possible word is used.

provider
(e.g., physicians, surgeons, advance practice nurses, physician's assistants) a licensed professional within scope of practice "who treats varying illnesses, prescribes medication to treat or cure illnesses, creates treatment plans and gives referrals when a treatment beyond their specialty is needed." (Best Accredited Colleges, 2022)

quality of life
(See HRQOL: Quality of Life)

serious illness
"a health condition that carries a high risk of mortality and either negatively impacts a person's daily function or quality of life or excessively strains their caregiver." (Kelley and Bollens-Lund, 2018)

serious illness trajectories
The course or progression of serious illness or disease as experienced over time. To date there are five trajectories (Barker &Scherer, 2016, Ballentine, 2018,).

shared decision-making
"A health care provider and a patient work together to make a health care decision that is best for the patient. The optimal decision takes into account evidence-based information about available options, the provider's knowledge and experience, and the patient's values and preferences" (AHRQ, 2016).

specialist palliative care
"Specialist palliative care is the active, total care of patients with serious illness and their families. Care is provided by an interdisciplinary team whose members have undergone recognized specialist palliative care training (NCP Guidelines, 2018, p.65).

spiritual/spirituality
"The aspect of humanity that refers to the way individuals seek and express meaning and purpose and the way they experience their connectedness to the moment, to self, to others, to nature, and to the significant or sacred" (NCP Guidelines, 2018. p. 65).

surrogate/proxy/health care agent
Known by other names, "is a substitute health-care decision-maker who consents or refuses to consent to some or all medical treatments for the patient who lacks decision-making capacity...Even when the patient appoints the surrogate, questions can still arise as to the extent of the surrogate's authority" (National POLST, 2022). An individual appointed to act on behalf of another when an individual is without capacity or has given permission (Law Insider, n.d.).

symptom management
"To prevent or treat as early as possible the symptoms of disease, side effects caused by treatment of a disease, and psychological, social, and spiritual problems related to a disease or its treatment" (Law Insider, n.d.). "Care given to help relieve the symptoms of a disease, such as cancer, and the side effects caused by treatment of the disease. Symptom management may help a person feel more comfortable, but it does not treat or cure the disease." (National Cancer Institute, n.d.)

treatment/therapy
The attempted remediation of a health problem, usually following a diagnosis, the medical or surgical management of a patient (Pallipedia website, 2022).

Wellbeing
The positive aspects of a person's life (HRQOL), such as positive emotions and life satisfaction (Healthy People 2020, 2020)

References /Resources

Agency for Healthcare Research and Quality (AHRQ). (2016). *The SHARE approach: A model for shared decision-making - Fact sheet.* https://www.ahrq.gov/health-literacy/professional-training/shared-decision/tools/factsheet.html

Agency for Healthcare Research and Quality (AHRQ). (2018). *Care coordination*. https://www.ahrq.gov/ncepcr/care/coordination.html

Alberta Health Services (AHS) Edmonton Zone Palliative Care Program. (2019). E*dmonton symptom assessment system* – Revised (ESAS-r). https://www.albertahealthservices.ca/assets/info/peolc/if-peolc-ed-esasr-admin-manual.pdf

American Medical Association (AMA). (2001). *Collaborative care (Opinion 10.8).* In Chapter 10 in AMA Medical Code of Ethics. https://code-medical-ethics.ama-assn.org/ethics-opinions/collaborative-care

American Medical Association (AMA). (2022). D*efining basic health care.* https://www.ama-assn.org/delivering-care/ethics/defining-basic-health-care

Ashkenazy, S., & DeKeyser Ganz, F. (2019). The differentiation between pain and discomfort: A concept analysis of discomfort. *Pain Manag Nurs*. 20(6), 556-562. doi:10.1016/j.pmn.2019.05.003

Ballentine, J.M. (2018). *The five trajectories: Supporting patients during serious illness.* Published by the CSU Shiley Institute for Palliative Care. https://csupalliativecare.org/wp-content/uploads/Five-Trajectories-eBook-02.21.2018.pdf

Baktari, J. (August 20, 2021). *DNR orders can lead to worse care & increase death rates*. https://www.e7health.com/articles/6/dnr-orders-can-lead-to-worse-care-increase-death-rates/

Barker, P.C. & Scherer, J.S. (2016). *Fast Fact #326- Illness trajectories: Description and clinical use.* Palliative Care Network of Wisconsin (PCNOW). https://www.mypcnow.org/fast-fact/illness-trajectories-description-and-clinical-use/

Barstow, C., Shahan, B., & Roberts, M. (2018). Evaluating medical decision-making capacity in *Am Fam Physician*, 98(1), 40-46.

Best Accredited Colleges. (October 20, 2021). *Difference between clinician & physician*. https://bestaccreditedcolleges.org/articles/difference-between-clinician-physician.html

Bock, A. (2022). *Serious Illness Messaging Toolkit*. https://www.seriousillnessmessaging.org/

Bruera, E., Kuehn, N., Miller, M.J., Selmser, P., &Macmillan, K. (1991). The Edmonton Symptom Assessment System (ESAS): a simple method of the assessment of palliative care patients. *Journal of Palliative Care* 1991; 7:6-9. *https://pubmed.ncbi.nlm.nih.gov/1714502/*

Center to Advance Palliative Care (CAPC). (May 15, 2023). *Introduction to palliative care for health professionals*. https://www.capc.org/training/introduction-to-palliative-care-for-health-professionals/

Center to Advance Palliative Care (CAPC). (November 26, 2019). *The case for improving communication and symptom management skills.* https://www.capc.org/documents/699/?utm_source=Center+to+Advance+Palliative+Care&utm_campaign=98e89c5623-The+Case+x3+10.4.22&utm_medium=email&utm_term=0_31106acbde-98e89c5623-369207313

Center to Advance Palliative Care (CAPC). (n.d.) *About palliative care.* https://www.capc.org/about/palliative-care/

Center for Disease Control and Prevention. (October 31, 2018). *HRQOL concepts*. https://archive.cdc.gov/#/details?url=https://www.cdc.gov/hrqol/concept.htm

Cleveland Clinic. (n.d.). *Life support*. https://my.clevelandclinic.org/health/treatments/12362-life-support-measures

Coelho, A., Parola, V., Escobar-Bravo, M. & Apostolo, J. (2016). Comfort experience in palliative care: A phenomenological study. *BMC Palliat Care* 15: 71. https://bmcpalliatcare.biomedcentral.com/articles/10.1186/s12904-016-0145-0

Davis, M.P & Hui, D. (2017). Quality of life in palliative care. *Expert Rev Qual Life Cancer Care.* 2(6):293-302. doi: 10.1080/23809000.2017.1400911. Epub 2017 Nov 8. PMID: 30854466; PMCID: PMC6405258. https://www.ncbi.nlm.nih.gov/pmc/articles/PMC6405258/#:~:text=Palliative%20care%20plays%20an%20important,realistic%20expectations%20through%20impeccable%20communication.

Ekberg, S., Parry, R., Land, V. et al. (2021). Communicating with patients and families about illness progression and end of life: A review of studies using direct observation of clinical practice. *BMC Palliat Care* 20:186-198. https://doi.org/10.1186/s12904-021-00876-2.

Getpalliativecare.org (August 11, 2023). *Four "C"s can help you understand palliative care*. https://getpalliativecare.org/four-cs-can-help-you-understand-palliative-care2023/

Given, B.A. & Reinhard, S.C. (2017). Caregiving at the end of life: The challenges for family caregivers. *Generations* 41:50–57. https://www.proquest.com/openview/99f5f726c76991721114210 2d2676520/1?pq-origsite=gscholar&cbl=30306

Goldish, A., & Rosielle, D. A. (2018). *Fast fact #365: Language for routine code status discussions*. https://www.mypcnow.org/fast-fact/language-for-routine-code-status-discussions/

Healthy People.gov/Healthy People 2020. (February 6, 2022). *Health-related quality of life and well-being.* https://www.healthypeople.

gov/2020/about/foundation-health-measures/Health-Related-Quality-of-Life-and-Well-Being

Hospice Foundation of America. (n.d.) *What is hospice?* https://hospicefoundation.org/Hospice-Care/Hospice-Services

International Association for Hospice & Palliative Care (IAHPC). (2022). *Allow natural death order (AND).* https://pallipedia.org/allow-natural-death-order-and/

Institute for Patient- and Family-Centered Care. (n.d.). *Patient and family centered care defined.* https://www.ipfcc.org/bestpractices/sustainable-partnerships/background/pfcc-defined.html

Joint Commission, The. (2018). *Comfort measures only. Specifications Manual for Joint Commission National Quality Measures (v2018A).* https://manual.jointcommission.org/releases/TJC2018A/DataElem0031.html

Kelley, A. S., & Bollens-Lund, E. (2018). Identifying the population with serious illness: The "denominator" challenge. *J Palliat Med*, 21(S2), S7-S16. Doi:10.1089/jpm.2017.0548

Law Insider (n.d.) *Surrogate decision maker definition*. https://www.lawinsider.com/dictionary/surrogate-decision-maker

Law Insider. (n.d.) *Medical treatment definition*. https://www.lawinsider.com/dictionary/medical-treatment

Law Insider. (n.d.). *Symptom management definition*. https://www.lawinsider.com/dictionary/symptom-management

McCaffery, M., & University of California, Los Angeles. (1968). *Nursing practice theories related to cognition, bodily pain, and man-environment interactions*. UCLA Students' Store.

National Cancer Institute at the National Institutes of Health. (n.d.). *Advance directive*. https://www.cancer.gov/publications/dictionaries/cancer-terms/def/advance-directive

National Cancer Institute/NIH. (n.d.). *Diagnosis*. ttps://www.cancer.gov/publications/dictionaries/cancer-terms/def/diagnosis

National Cancer Institute/NIH. (n.d.). *Standard medical care.* https://www.cancer.gov/publications/dictionaries/cancer-terms/def/standard-medical-care

National Consensus Project for Quality Palliative Care/National Coalition for Hospice and Palliative Care (NCP Guidelines). (2018). Clinician definition. In *Clinical Practice Guidelines for Quality Palliative Care (4th Ed.).* https://www.nationalcoalitionhpc.org/wp-content/uploads/2020/07/NCHPC-NCPGuidelines_4thED_web_FINAL.pdf

- Quality of life, p. 13
- Care Coordination, p. 60
- Clinician definition, p. 61
- Communication definition, p. 61
- Primary palliative care, p. 64
- Specialist palliative care, p. 65
- Spirituality definition, p. 65

National POLST. (2022). *Understanding advance care planning.* https://polst.org/advance-care-plans

National POLST. (2018). *Advance care planning: Surrogates.* http://polst.org/wp-content/uploads/2018/03/2018.03.01-Surrogate-Definition-and-Role-in-Advance-Care-Planning.pdf

National POLST. (2022). *POLST: Honoring the wishes of those with serious illness and frailty.* https://polst.org/

NEJM Catalyst. (January 1, 2017). *What is Patient-Centered Care?* https://catalyst.nejm.org/doi/full/10.1056/CAT.17.0559

Nelson, C. M., & Nazareth, B. A. (2013). Nonbeneficial treatment and conflict resolution: building consensus. *The Permanenteournal*, 17(3), 23–27. https://doi.org/10.7812/TPP/12-124

North Dakota Palliative Care Taskforce. (January 2020). *Palliative care or hospice care?* https://ruralhealth.und.edu/assets/746-17373/palliative-hospice-care-flyer.pdf

Odden, A. & Dastidar, J. G. (August 3, 2011). *How do I determine if my patient has decision-making capacity?* https://www.the-hospitalist.org/hospitalist/article/124731/how-do-i-determine-if-my-patient-has-decision-making-capacity

Pallipedia The Free Online Palliative Care Dictionary. (2022).

- *Allow Natural Death.* https://pallipedia.org/allow-natural-death-order-and/
- *End of Life Care.* https://pallipedia.org/end-of-life-care/
- *Hope.* https://pallipedia.org/hope/
- *Goals of Care: What does it mean?* https://pallipedia.org/goals-of-care-what-does-it-mean/
- *Prognosis.* https://pallipedia.org/prognosis/
- *Quality of Life in Palliative Care:* https://pallipedia.org/quality-of-life-in-palliative-care/
- *Quality of Medical Care.* https://pallipedia.org/quality-of-medical-care/

Pantilat, S. (2018). *Why palliative care is essential in the face of serious illness.* TedMed. https://www.tedmed.com/talks/show?id=731059

Parker, J. (June 27, 2022). *The case for integrating social determinants into palliative care.* Hospice News. https://hospicenews.com/2022/06/27/the-case-for-integrating-social-determinants-into-palliative-care/

Parker, J. (January 10, 2020). *Palliative care well-poised to address social determinants of health*. Hospice News. https://hospicenews.com/2020/01/10/palliative-care-well-poised-to-address-social-determinants-of-health/

Paulson, D. S. (2004). Taking care of patients and caring for patients are not the same. AORN J, 79(2), 359-62, 365-6. doi:10.1016/s0001-2092(06)60612-1

Pottash, M. (2018). *Fast fact #365: Language for routine code status discussions*. https://www.pallimed.org/2019/05/comfort-care-whatever-does-that-mean_4.html

Prabhakar, A. & Smith, T. J. (2021). *Fast fact #417: Total pain*. https://www.mypcnow.org/fast-fact/total-pain/

Sudore, R. L., Lum, H. D., You, J. J., Hanson, L. C., Meier, D. E., Pantilat, S. Z., Matlock, D. D., Rietjens, J. A. C., Korfage, I. J., Ritchie, C. S., Kutner, J.S., Teno, J. M., Thomas, J., McMahan, R. D., & Heyland, D. K. (2017). Defining advance care planning for adults: A consensus definition from a multidisciplinary Delphi panel. *J Pain Symptom Manage*, 53(5):821-832.el. doi:10.1016/j.jpainsymman.2016.12.331

Vitas Health Care. (n.d.). *Hospice & palliative care definitions*. https://www.vitas.com/hospice-and-palliative-care-basics/about-hospice-care/hospice-glossary

World Health Organization.(2022). *Social determinants of health*. https://www.who.int/health-topics/social-determinants-of-health#tab=tab_1

Zolkefli, Y. (2017). Evaluating the Concept of Choice in Healthcare. *Malays J Med Sci*. 24(6):92-96. doi: 10.21315/mjms2017.24.6.11. Epub 2017 Dec 29. PMID: 29379391; PMCID: PMC5771520. https://www.ncbi.nlm.nih.gov/pmc/articles/PMC5771520/#:~:text=Giving%20patients%20choices%20has%20been,choices%2C%20values%2C%20and%20needs

Diagram: The 4 Cs of Palliative Care

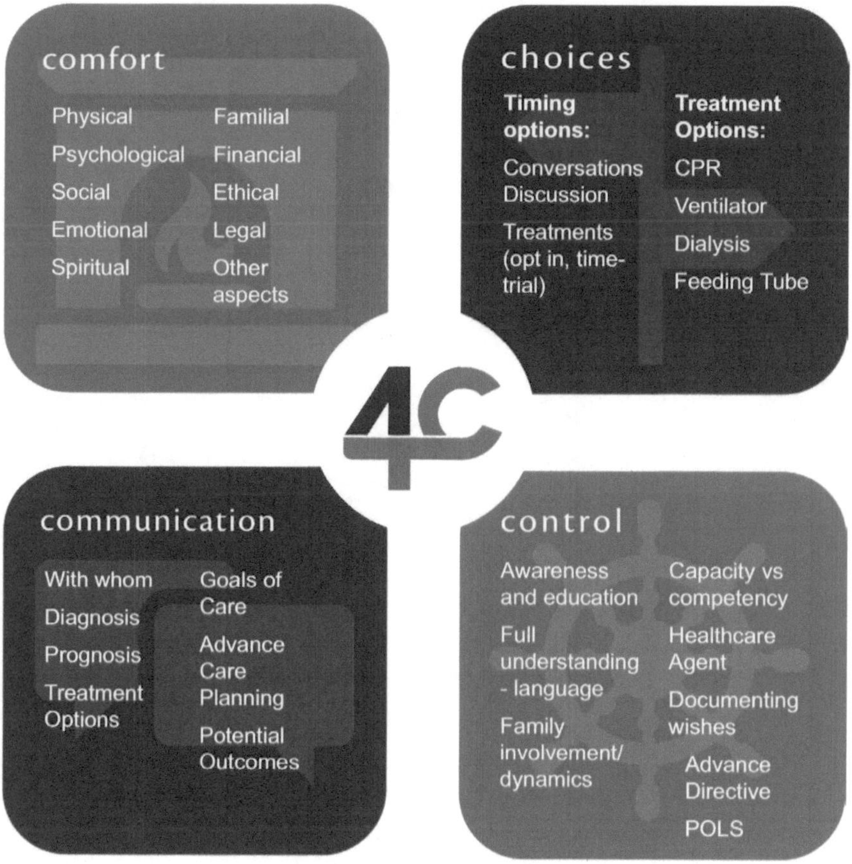